TRAUMA RULES

Edited by

TIM HODGETTS MRCP (UK), FFAEM,
DiplMC RCSEd, RAMC

*Consultant, Accident and Emergency Medicine,
Ministry of Defence Hospital Unit, Frimley Park, Camberley,
Surrey, UK*

STEPHEN DEANE FRACS, FRCSC, FACS

*Professor of Surgery, University of New South Wales and
Liverpool Hospital, Sydney, Australia*

KEITH GUNNING FRCS(Ed)

General and Trauma Surgeon, Newcastle, UK

BMJ
Publishing
Group

© BMJ Publishing Group 1997

First published in 1997
by the BMJ Publishing Group, BMA House,
Tavistock Square, London WC1H 9JR

British Library Cataloguing in Publication Data

A catalogue record for this book is available
from the British Library

ISBN 0–7279–1148–1

Typeset, printed and bound in Great Britain by
Latimer Trend and Company Ltd, Plymouth

Contents

Investigation and definitive care

Contributors

Professor Ken Hillman, Intensive Care Specialist, Liverpool, New South Wales, Australia

Stuart Matthews, Orthopaedic and Trauma Surgeon, Leeds, UK

Professor Peter Roberts, Surgeon, Royal Army Medical Corps, UK

Maria Seger, Trauma Nurse Consultant, Liverpool, New South Wales, Australia

Michael Sugrue, Surgeon, Director of Trauma, Liverpool, New South Wales, Australia

Foreword

The management of major trauma may seem to be a complex issue but it can be approached in a systematic manner. This book combines a systematic approach with a novel series of *trauma rules* to trigger the memory when faced with a seriously injured patient.

Each rule is accompanied by the reason, the exceptions to the rule and, where appropriate, an illustration highlighting a key aspect of the rule.

Learning should be fun, and this book is designed to be fun to read. It is hoped that these *trauma rules* may be used by those involved in trauma education at all professional levels to emphasise the key issues in trauma management and to perpetuate a high standard of trauma care.

Trauma Rules is an *aide-mémoire* and supplements existing textbooks on this subject. Readers who require a more extensive understanding of the management of trauma are referred to the following books, also published by BMJ Publishing Group.

- *ABC of Major Trauma*
- *Trauma: Beyond the resuscitation room*

Tim Hodgetts
Stephen Deane
Keith Gunning

London and Sydney

Rules are made to be broken,
That's not what you should do.
For one of these days these rules
Will help you save a life or two.

Approach
to the
patient

Anxiety provokes memory loss: so learn a system and stick to it

The reason

When the chips are down you may only have your own experience to rely on. When your experience is limited you need rules that are easy to remember and easy to apply, even in the most threatening of circumstances. This system is:

Airway, with control of the cervical spine;
Breathing, with oxygen; and
Circulation, with control of external blood loss.

This **ABC** system allows the identification and treatment of life-threatening injuries in a rapid, logical and reproducible order. The patient assessment is extended to include:

Disability (neurological status) and
Exposure, with Environmental considerations (control of body temperature).

Together, the initial patient assessment following this **ABCDE** system is known as the "primary survey". This is the systematic approach taught on the internationally established *Advanced Trauma Life Support* course[1] (adapted as the *Early Management of Severe Trauma* course in Australia) and *Pre-hospital Trauma Life Support* course.[2]

The exceptions

To the beginner in trauma management, there are no exceptions to this rule. This is your code of practice. The experienced clinician, however, will regard all rules as guidelines – but will still closely follow **ABC** principles.

[1]American College of Surgeons. *Advanced Trauma Life Support Provider Manual.* 1993.
[2]National Association of Emergency Medical Technicians. *Pre-hospital Trauma Life Support*, 3rd edn, Mosby Lifeline, 1994.

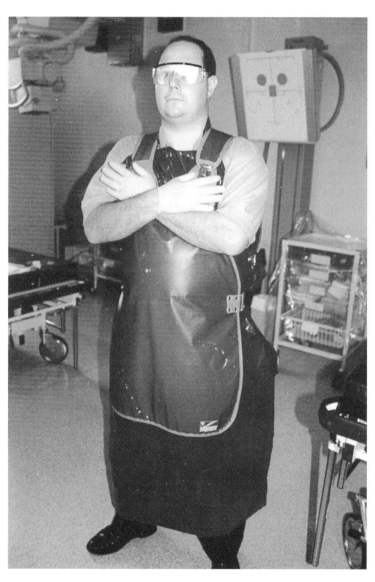

Save yourself before the casualty.

Save yourself before the casualty

The reason

All trauma patients should be considered a high risk for blood transmissible diseases, particularly the HIV, hepatitis B, and hepatitis C viruses. If you as a health care worker have an infection with one of these viruses you have an ethical, and in some cases a legal, responsibility to declare this, or remove yourself from the environment where you may come into contact with the injured.

Remember:

> *Think of your safety to begin,*
> *When infected you're no use to him.*

Personal protective equipment for the resuscitation room should include:

- Eye protection (goggles/safety glasses/visor/face-shield)
- Impervious gown or apron
- Latex gloves
- Lead apron

When there is advanced warning, the team should be appropriately dressed before the patient arrives.

The exceptions

It is easy to think of the situation when a seriously injured patient arrives at hospital and the staff have not had time to protect themselves adequately. This is no excuse. ALWAYS take suitable precautions to protect yourself from a patient's bodily fluids before you give treatment.

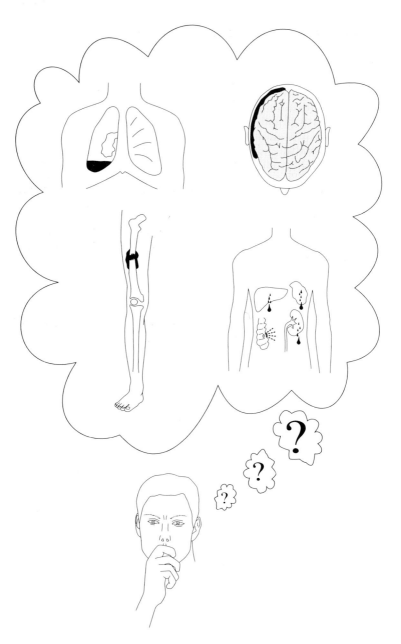

Assume the worst and proceed accordingly.

Assume the worst and proceed accordingly

The reason

Every patient who fulfills the criteria to activate the trauma team should be treated in the same manner. Do not be tempted to take short-cuts in the primary survey.

The disadvantage of adopting a rigid protocol for all trauma victims is that a proportion will be overtreated, will have undergone invasive procedures (venous cannulation, rectal and vaginal examination, urinary catheterisation) and will have been exposed to radiation without any significant injury being discovered. Some may even be discharged home from the resuscitation room. This is the price for not missing those who do have significant but initially occult injury, suggested by the mechanism of injury rather than the anatomical injury or the physiological signs at the scene of injury.

The exceptions

Only substantial clinical experience in trauma management can justify any short-cuts to the assessment and treatment of trauma victims.

Do a frisk or take a risk

The reason

Do not assume that a patient who has been shot or stabbed is an innocent victim of an unprovoked crime. There may have been a two-way exchange of violence.

Hypoxia causes confusion and aggression. Do not give the hypoxic patient the opportunity of confusing you with an aggressor. Do a rapid frisk for weapons and make them safe. If you do not know how to make a firearm safe, place it on the floor out of the way and have it guarded until the police arrive.

The exceptions

An armed assailant who has been injured during apprehension by the police will already have been frisked for weapons.

Don't let the obvious distract from the occult

The reason

An immediately obvious injury may distract you from a less obvious but life-threatening injury. This is particularly likely with orthopaedic injuries – for example a large joint dislocation or angulated long-bone fracture will immediately attract your attention, but will you immediately notice the obstructed airway or tension pneumothorax?

For this reason, it is always wise to follow the ABC approach to assessment and management of an injured patient.

The exceptions

Some obvious injuries are life-threatening, for example a traumatic limb amputation with arterial haemorrhage. However, it is still recommended to follow the ABC approach, even if assessment of airway and breathing is rapid and the management of A and B is confined to the administration of high-concentration oxygen. This concept may be difficult to accept in the face of exsanguinating external haemorrhage, but remember that a trauma team often works "horizontally", with airway, breathing and circulation being assessed and managed simultaneously (if you are on your own you must work "vertically" and attend to A then B then C).

The trauma team can only look or listen, not both

The reason

It is a common observation that the trauma team fail to absorb the information from the ambulance paramedic during the hand-over of the patient. This is because the human being is essentially a single channel processor, and the doctor who is concentrating on assessing the patient cannot also concentrate on the spoken information from the paramedic.

One way to address this problem is for the whole trauma team to stand and listen to the patient hand-over before anyone approaches the patient. The paramedic is given up to 45 seconds to describe:

M   Mechanism of injury
I   Injuries found and suspected
S   Signs (respiratory rate, oxygen saturation, pulse rate, blood pressure)
T   Treatment given

This is time well spent: it will reduce unnecessary repetition of the story and will prevent vital information being lost. It is useful to have a board in the resuscitation room on which to write this information, placed where anyone else entering the room can see it.

The exceptions

The trauma team will not wait for a hand-over if basic life support is in progress, or if the airway is obstructed. In this case, the team leader should instruct the ambulance crew to wait for an opportunity to pass the pre-hospital information.

Initial assessment and resuscitation

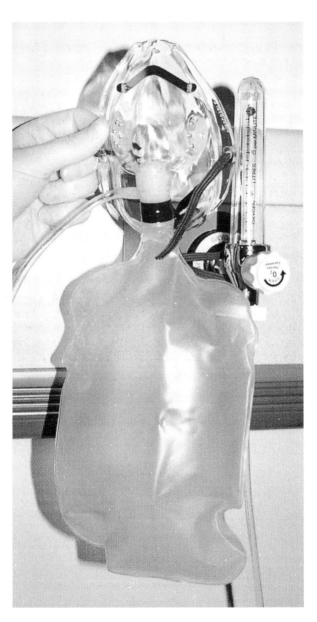

All trauma patients are dying for oxygen.

All trauma patients are dying for oxygen

The reason

All victims of significant trauma will have a degree of hypoxia as a result of either airway compromise, chest injury, hypoventilation from head injury, or hypovolaemia. To improve oxygen delivery to hypoxic tissues, all victims of trauma should be given high-concentration oxygen. When spontaneously breathing, the best delivery system is a tight-fitting Hudson face-mask with an attached reservoir bag and oxygen at 10–15 l/min, adjusted to the minimum flow required to keep the reservoir bag inflated. This provides an inspired oxygen concentration in excess of 85% ($FiO_2 > 0.85$).

If ventilation is being assisted, 100% oxygen can be delivered through a bag-valve device (attached to a mask or endotracheal tube) when a reservoir bag is incorporated into the system and the oxygen flow is adjusted between 10 and 15 l/min to keep the reservoir inflated.

The exceptions

It is essential to give all victims of significant trauma supplemental high-concentration oxygen, even those patients with chronic lung disease. They are all hypoxic, and hypoxia is compounded if there is chronic lung disease. If respiration is suppressed, ventilation can be assisted. Remember: CO_2 kills slowly, but no O_2 kills quickly.

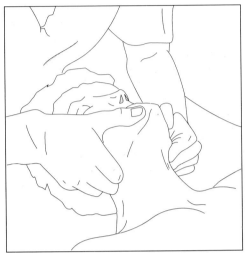

Jaw thrust to open the airway (the preferred manoeuvre following trauma).

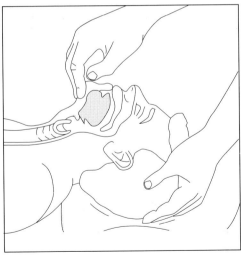

Head tilt plus chin lift to open the airway.

The airway is more important than the cervical spine

The reason

The judgement to immobilise the cervical spine is often based on the mechanism of injury rather than the presence of symptoms and signs indicating spinal injury. The cervical spine is therefore usually immobilised because of **potential** injury, not absolute injury. However, airway obstruction is an **absolute** problem: if untreated the patient will certainly die.

In general, the airway is opened and secured while stabilising the cervical spine. To assist intubation, the hard collar may be removed while manual in-line stabilisation is maintained. But when there is impending death from airway obstruction protection of the cervical spine may be overlooked.[1] This may include tilting the head to obtain a clear airway.

The exceptions

Even in the presence of clinical signs of spinal injury, the airway **must** take first priority. In any case, the patient who most benefits from immobilisation is the one **without** neurological symptoms. If there are symptoms, the damage has been done already and is unlikely to be made worse by the pre-hospital handling or handling in the resuscitation room.

[1]Lewis FR, Trunkey DD. Emergency department care. In: Trunkey DD, Lewis FR, eds. *Current therapy of trauma 1984–85*. Philadelphia: BC Decker, 1984.

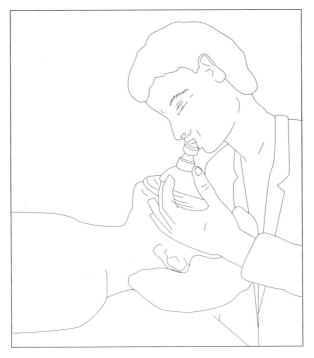

Ventilation via a pocket mask.
Do not overlook the simple ventilation techniques.

It is not lack of intubation that kills, it is lack of oxygenation

The reason

Assisted ventilation may be required because of *hypoventilation* (as a result of the injury or respiratory depressant drugs, such as opiates used for analgesia), because of *ineffective ventilation* (for example with a flail chest and underlying contusion) or in *traumatic cardiac arrest.*

A bag-valve mask is often sufficient in the pre-hospital or early hospital resuscitation phases to provide oxygenation. Intubation can only be attempted in the pre-hospital setting when the patient is completely unresponsive, as generally there is no access to intravenous anaesthetic and paralysing agents. Should intubation be attempted outside hospital, it is important that the patient is pre-oxygenated before each attempt and that professional pride does not prevent the crew reverting to a simpler technique. Equally, the bag-valve mask technique can be difficult with one operator (two operators are ideal, with one to hold the mask with both hands and one to ventilate) and the operator should not be afraid to discard the bag-valve mask in favour of a Laerdal Pocket Mask™. It is better to deliver 17% expired air oxygen to the lungs than to deliver 100% oxygen to the back of the mouth.

The Laryngeal Mask Airway and the Combi-tube are advanced airway adjuncts that can be positioned blind (without the need for a laryngoscope) by medical, paramedical, or nursing staff after relatively little training. The devices allow ventilation via a bag-valve device, but in general do not provide the same degree of airway protection as a cuffed endotracheal tube. Their use is becoming increasingly popular in the emergency situation.

The exceptions

A patient with a head injury who is comatose (Glasgow Coma Scale <9) on arrival at hospital requires early endotracheal intubation to protect the airway, to provide a reliable route of supplying high-concentration oxygen to limit secondary brain damage, and to hyperventilate the patient to lower the partial pressure of carbon dioxide where appropriate. In this case, it is reasonable to aim for intubation within ten minutes of arrival in the resuscitation room. It is vital to preoxygenate the patient before each intubation attempt. Should the oesophagus be intubated, this is not negligent – it is only negligent to fail to recognise it has occurred.

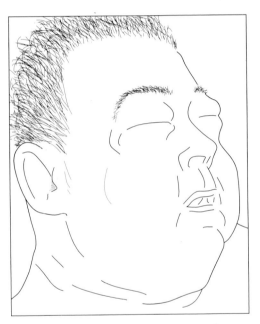

Anticipate obstruction of the airway with facial oedema following burns.
Do not delay with a burned airway.

Do not delay with a burned airway

The reason

Laryngeal oedema secondary to inhalational burns develops very rapidly, often within minutes, and can present the anaesthetist with one of the most difficult intubations they are likely to face. The following signs indicate the presence of upper airway burns and the need to consider early elective intubation:

- Respiratory distress
- Burns around the mouth
- Oedema of the face or lips
- Oropharyngeal carbon or carbonaceous sputum
- Singed nasal hairs
- Inflammation, oedema, or blistering of the oropharynx or tongue
- Hoarse voice

When there are inhalational burns, always consider concomitant carbon-monoxide poisoning. The principal treatment is high-concentration oxygen. Hyperbaric oxygen should be considered in the following circumstances:

- Loss of consciousness at scene
- Carboxyhaemoglobin levels >30%*
- Pregnancy
- Presence of focal neurological signs

*This threshold may vary between hyperbaric units and should be checked locally.

The exceptions

Flash burns will often cause superficial burns and singeing of the eyebrows and hair, but may not involve the upper airway. Look for the suggestive signs of additional upper airway burn listed above.

While hyperbaric oxygen will greatly reduce the half-life of carboxyhaemoglobin (to about 20 minutes), the benefit of this treatment must be balanced against the need for other life-saving treatment, such as surgery for injuries incurred during an escape from the fire. The hyperbaric unit may be no more than a coffin-sized chamber and, if complications arise during treatment, intervention to treat them can be difficult. If the patient requires an endotracheal tube the cuff should be filled with water, otherwise it will deflate and the tube may become dislodged.

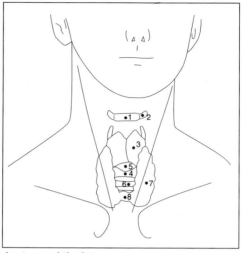

Anatomy of the larynx

1. Body of hyoid cartilage
2. Greater horn of hyoid cartilage
3. Thyroid cartilage
4. Cricoid cartilage
5. Cricothyroid membrane
6. Tracheal ring
7. Lobe of thyroid
8. Thyroid isthmus

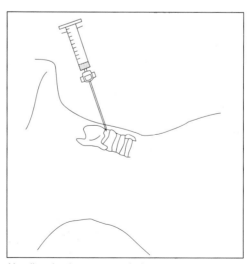

Needle cricothyrotomy technique.

Think of cricothyrotomy when all else fails

The reason

Cricothyrotomy is a means of bypassing an obstructed upper airway when all other means of obtaining an airway have failed, including manual manoeuvres (chin lift or jaw thrust), simple airway adjuncts (oropharyngeal and nasopharyngeal), and endotracheal intubation.

Cricothyrotomy may be necessary in the resuscitation room with upper airway obstruction secondary to a foreign body or oedema (from burns, facial fractures or, rarely, anaphylaxis from drugs administered).

A *needle cricothyrotomy* involves inserting a large bore cannula through the cricothyroid membrane and jet-insufflating oxygen from a cylinder or wall source. A *surgical circothyrotomy* requires an incision in the cricothyroid membrane through which a tracheostomy-type tube can be inserted. The minimal definitive airway for an adult is 6 mm internal diameter.

A principal complication is to insert the needle or the tube anterior to the membrane, subcutaneously. When assisted ventilation is started, the neck will distend with massive surgical emphysema and landmarks will be lost.

The exceptions

In children under 12 years, a surgical cricothyrotomy is not recommended. This is because the tracheal cartilage rings are immature and the support for the upper trachea is provided by the cricoid cartilage. When the cricothyroid membrane is incised this support can be lost.

A tracheostomy is not a technique for the emergency room. It requires a skilled surgeon, is more time consuming, and has a considerable risk of significant haemorrhage.

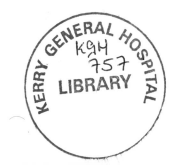

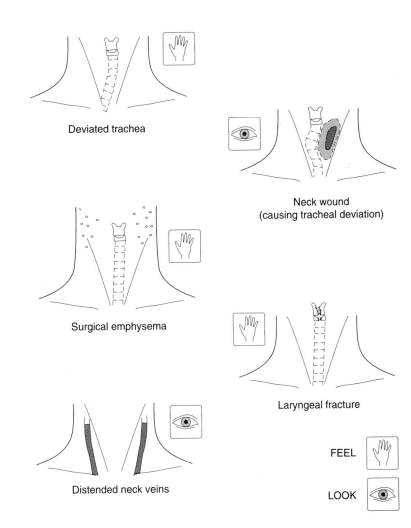

Deviated trachea

Neck wound
(causing tracheal deviation)

Surgical emphysema

Laryngeal fracture

Distended neck veins

FEEL

LOOK

Look at the neck six times in the primary survey.

Look at the neck six times in the primary survey

The reason

The neck carries the airway and the circulation to the brain. For this reason it is important to examine the neck in the primary survey. It is natural to do this after inspecting the upper airway and before examining the chest. The considerations are as follows:

Trachea	If this is deviated, suspect a tension pneumothorax.
Wounds	Are there wounds in the neck threatening the airway or circulation? Do not probe these wounds in the emergency department.
Emphysema	Surgical emphysema in the neck may suggest a disrupted airway or a pneumothorax.
Larynx	Is the larynx intact? If not, the airway is in immediate danger.
Veins	Distended neck veins suggest a tension pneumothorax or cardiac tamponade.
Every time	DON'T FORGET to look at the neck before you put on the hard collar. With the collar in place you may miss these important signs.

The exceptions

A hard cervical collar is usually in place when a trauma victim arrives at hospital, often with additional cervical spine support. Many hard collars still allow limited examination of the neck through a cut-away section anteriorly. Unless there is a suspicion of a life-threatening injury in the neck, the collar should not be removed routinely in the primary survey but will be removed as part of the secondary survey while maintaining manual immobilisation of the cervical spine.

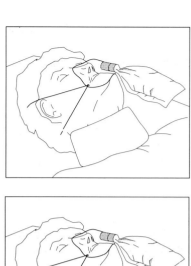

Soft collar

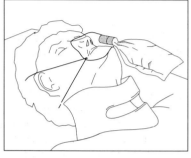

Hard collar

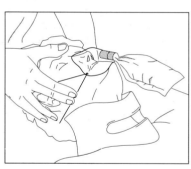

Hard collar and hands

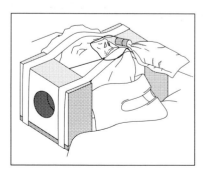

Hard collar and head box

A hard collar does not protect the cervical spine

The reason

A soft collar does not protect the cervical spine – it will simply keep the neck warm. A hard collar is just a flag which says, "Protect this neck, it may be injured", and on its own it is also inadequate protection for the cervical spine. A hard collar must be paired with manual in-line stabilisation or rigid head immobilisation (in a head-box, or with sandbags and tape).

Following blunt multi-system trauma, the cervical spine should be assumed to be injured until this has been excluded radiologically and clinically. A high index of suspicion is particularly important with significant other injury above the clavicle.

At the cervical level, the spinal cord occupies about 50% of the spinal canal, the rest of the space being filled with connective tissue and fat. It is therefore possible to cause damage to the cervical spine and narrowing of the canal without causing neurological impairment. Careless handling of the patient during extrication and resuscitation could cause further narrowing and precipitate quadraplegia. Remember that it is the patient **without** neurological symptoms who will benefit most from rigid spinal immobilisation in the resuscitation.

The exceptions

If the patient is very agitated (and this is common in distressed children) it can be detrimental to rigidly immobilise the head, as the body continues to move. In these cases a collar alone has to suffice.

Penetrating trauma to the neck, such as from a gunshot wound, will produce neurological symptoms immediately following injury. If there are no symptoms, there is no injury.

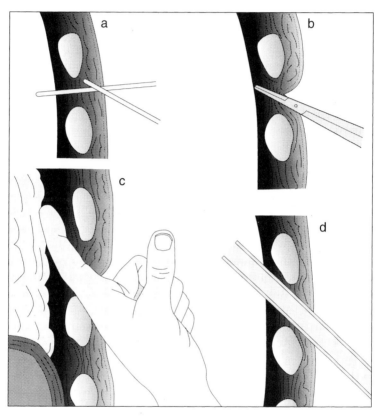

Chest drain insertion. (a) Penetration of the skin, muscle and pleura. (b) Blunt dissection of the intercostal muscles and penetration of the parietal pleura. (c) Exploration of the pleural cavities. (d) Tube (without trocar) directed posteriorly and superiorly.

All Trauma surgeons Occasionally Miss Cervical Fractures

The reason

There are six life-threatening chest conditions that must be considered following trauma. Each of these should be actively sought during the primary survey, and treated immediately when found. The conditions can be remembered as: "All Trauma surgeons Occasionally Miss Cervical Fractures".

All	Airway obstruction
Trauma surgeons	Tension pneumothorax
Occasionally	Open pneumothorax
Miss	Massive haemothorax
Cervical	Cardiac tamponade
Fractures	Flail chest

Only 10 to 15% of patients with blunt or penetrating chest injury require thoracotomy,[1] so 85 to 90% of chest injuries can be treated by a variable combination of observation, chest drainage, pain control, and respiratory support.

The exceptions

There are no exceptions to this rule for blunt trauma (a fall or a motor vehicle accident), but a clear mechanism of penetrating injury (such as a stab or gunshot wound) will not produce a flail chest.

Inserting a chest drain will treat tension pneumothorax, open pneumothorax, and massive haemothorax. However, the **immediate** treatment for each of these conditions is as follows:

Tension pneumothorax	–	Needle decompression
Open pneumothorax	–	Seal with watertight dressing on three sides
Massive haemothorax	–	Start fluids before chest drain

The main treatment for a flail chest is to treat the underlying contusion, which may require ventilatory support. A chest drain would be inserted for an accompanying pneumothorax, and may be appropriate prophylactically with multiple rib fractures before positive pressure ventilation (a small, unseen pneumothorax would otherwise tension).

---

[1]Kish G, Kozloll L, Joseph W, *et al*. Indications for early thoracotomy in the management of chest trauma. *Annals of Thoracic Surgery* 1976; **22**: 23.

Rule 15

When patients with facial injuries look up at heaven they will soon be there

The reason

Airway obstruction is the principal cause of death with facial injuries.[1]

With mid-face fractures (Le Fort fractures), the face may slide posteriorly along the incline of the base of the skull when the patient is supine. A conscious patient with an unstable mid-face will often adopt the most comfortable position for breathing, which is likely to be sitting up and leaning forward. In this position the airway is patent, but will become obstructed if the ambulance officer or resuscitation room physician insists on the patient lying flat.

When the patient is sitting it is important to immobilise the cervical spine in a hard collar – but maintaining the airway is more important than insisting on rigid cervical spinal immobilisation in the supine position (see Rule 8).

Airway obstruction with facial injuries may also be a result of heavy bleeding, or from the swelling associated with a fractured jaw.

The exceptions

A patient who is unconscious will be managed in the supine position. The airway can be maintained in the first-aid situation by rolling the patient into the recovery position, but at the risk of inadequately controlling the cervical spine. If the patient is managed in the supine position, the airway may be simply maintained by a combination of suction (to clear aspirated blood), traction on the upper incisors (to pull a shattered mid-face forward), or traction through a transverse tongue suture (when a severely disrupted jaw allows the tongue to fall back into the pharynx).

With a supine patient the cervical spine should be fully immobilised. There is a significant risk of concomitant cervical spine damage with any high-impact blunt injury above the clavicle.

[1]Kelly KF. *Management of war injuries to the jaw and related structures*. Washington, DC 1978. US Government Printing Office, Document 008.

Blood on the floor is forever lost to the patient

The reason

The priority in the treatment of circulation is to arrest external haemorrhage. Why attempt to replace something that you can prevent being lost? Bleeding wounds should therefore be dressed before, or at the same time as, intravenous access is obtained.

To make a rapid assessment for hidden but significant blood loss on the back of the supine patient, run gloved hands behind the chest and abdomen, and behind the legs. You will need to examine the back of the scalp in the secondary survey as blood loss from scalp wounds can be severe. Remember to look at the sheets and the canvas stretcher; significant blood loss may not have reached the floor.

The exceptions

Blood may not be lost forever when the facilities for autotransfusion ("cell saving") exist. This technique was first attempted in 1886 when Duncan reinfused the blood of a patient whose legs were crushed in a railway incident.

Blood may be outside the circulation for one to four hours and still be reinfused (through a micropore filter to remove any debris). A maximum of 3 litres of autotransfused blood is recommended, and as an adjunct to cross-matched blood. It is particularly valuable in massive haemothorax. The technique is less attractive for intra-abdominal bleeding because of the risk of bacterial contamination,[1] although it can be considered, when available, for isolated solid organ haemorrhage.

Overall, the advantages of autotransfusion are that the blood is immediately available and pre-warmed, there are no transfusion reactions, and the risk of blood-borne infection is eliminated. The disadvantages are air embolism (very rare in the latest systems), disseminated intravascular coagulopathy, and thrombocytopaenia.

The technique is not widely used in resuscitation rooms in the United Kingdom, perhaps through a combination of cost, absence of back-up technical staff, and a lack of familiarity.

---

[1]Gervin AS. Transfusion, autotransfusion, and blood substitutes. In Moore E, Mattox K, Feliciano D. *Trauma*. Connecticut: Appleton and Lange, 1991.

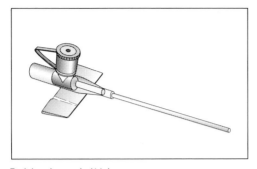

Peripheral cannula (14g).

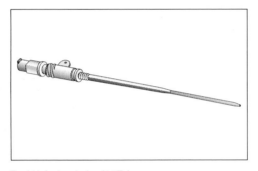

Rapid infusion device (7.5Fg).

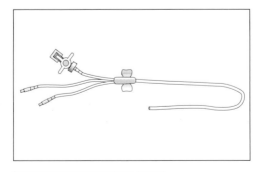

Central venous catheter (triple lumen).

Short and thick does the trick

The reason

Do not be fooled into thinking that the patient needs a central line for adequate fluid resuscitation. Flow through a tube is inversely proportional to its length and directly proportional to its radius (to the power four). Central lines are often long and thin, whereas peripheral lines are often short and thick. In particular, a "drum catheter" is a central line placed peripherally, usually in the antecubital fossa, and has a very long cannula.

In general, therefore, the patient is best served by fluid resuscitation through a large peripheral cannula. A 16 gauge cannula is not a large peripheral cannula: it is the lower limit of the large range and the minimum size for adequate fluid resuscitation.

The rapid infusion device is a good example of this principle. A short, wide-bore cannula ($\sim 6\cdot5$–$8\cdot0$ Fg) is inserted by percutaneous Seldinger technique (for example into the femoral vein), by "rewiring" an existing smaller peripheral cannula (for example an 18 g cannula in the forearm), or directly through an incision in the vein wall during a cutdown (for example the long saphenous vein).

Remember, flow is not only dependent on the length and radius of the cannula but also on the viscosity, temperature, and pressure of the fluid:

$$\text{Flow} = \frac{P\pi r^4}{8\eta L}$$

where
P = pressure difference
r = radius of the cannula
η = viscosity of the fluid
L = length of the cannula

The exceptions

A Swan–Ganz catheter sheath is placed centrally, usually in the internal jugular vein, but it does have a wide diameter and can be very effective for fluid resuscitation. It should only be inserted by an experienced person, generally an anaesthetist or intensive care specialist.

Rule 18

Hidden blood loss will CRAMP your resuscitation

The reason

Signs of blood loss without obvious external haemorrhage include pallor and sweating, tachycardia, tachypnoea, narrow pulse pressure or hypotension, and reduced urinary output. Continuing blood loss is suggested by a failure to respond to intravenous fluid challenges or a non-sustained response.

The following sites of hidden blood loss should be excluded:

C	Chest	Do a chest radiograph
R	Retroperitoneum	Test the urine
A	Abdomen	Do a diagnostic peritoneal lavage
M	Missed long-bone fracture	Examine the limbs
P	Pelvis	Do a pelvic radiograph

To discover a haemothorax that is not clinically obvious, a chest radiograph is obtained after the primary survey. To determine if there is retroperitoneal bleeding, the urine is examined for macroscopic or microscopic blood. Macroscopic blood requires further investigation (structural changes are best seen on a CT scan, whereas function is best seen on an intravenous urogram). Intra-abdominal bleeding is suggested by tenderness, distension, guarding, and rigidity. When intra-abdominal injury is suspected but the signs are equivocal, a diagnostic peritoneal lavage should be performed. A long-bone fracture may be missed when the patient is unresponsive or when a spinal cord injury has produced a loss of sensation. These fractures will be detected by careful clinical examination. Equally, a pelvic fracture may be missed in these circumstances, and a pelvic radiograph should also be obtained after the primary survey.

The exceptions

It is also important to consider that external blood loss at the scene may have been underestimated, and that an inadequate response to fluid replacement may simply mean inadequate fluid replacement when there is no continuing blood loss. A severe scalp wound would be a good example (see Rule 16).

Surgery does not follow resuscitation, it is part of resuscitation

The reason

A man with a hole in his bath does not keep pouring in water to keep the bath full; he plugs the hole. Similarly, a patient with an exsanguinating injury requires surgery, not just an endless supply of intravenous fluids. The aim of intravenous fluids in this circumstance is to sustain the patient until life-saving surgery can be performed.

The trauma patient who is "too ill for surgery" will surely die without surgery. It is not appropriate to wait for surgery until a target pulse or blood pressure is reached with intravenous fluids; in some cases this will never be achieved. However, all measures should be taken to try to ensure the patient is adequately volume resuscitated before emergency surgery.

In certain circumstances, there is now both experimental and clinical data to show that aggressive fluid resuscitation before surgery can even be harmful. Specifically, people with penetrating torso injuries have been shown to fare better when fluid resuscitation is delayed until the operating room.

The exceptions

A patient who is moved from the emergency department without their airway being secured, without adequate intravenous access, and without a supply of intravenous fluids is very vulnerable on the journey to the operating theatre. Although emergency surgery is part of resuscitation, it does not replace the need to start other resuscitative measures in the emergency department.

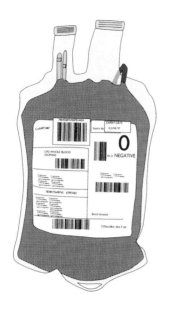

IS

GOOD

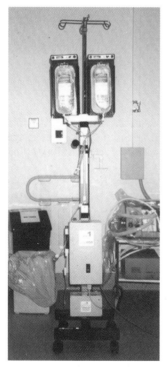

ALL
BLOOD
SHOULD
BE
WARM

O Negative is good, but you can have too much of a good thing

The reason

O Rhesus Negative blood is regarded as the universal donor group. Hospitals will keep a small supply of this blood group for emergency administration of untyped blood. This should be reserved for immediately life-threatening haemorrhage that cannot be stabilised with colloid for the ten to fifteen minutes it takes to obtain type-specific blood.

If more than four units of O Rhesus Negative blood is given, then there will be an admixture of blood cells of different groups. This would interfere with any subsequent cross-match. The sample for cross-match would, however, usually be taken on insertion of the intravenous cannula and before any blood is given.

If more than four units of O Rhesus Negative blood are given to a non-O patient who then receives a transfusion of their own blood type, there is likely to be a major haemolytic transfusion reaction.[1]

Do not give more than four units of O Rhesus Negative blood without knowing the patient's blood group.

The exceptions

If the patient's blood group is O Rhesus Negative, then you should continue to administer this blood group.

O Rhesus Negative blood will only rarely be required in trauma resuscitation, for those patients with critical hypovolaemia (more than 40% blood volume lost) who do not respond to colloid alone in the ten to fifteen minutes it takes to obtain type-specific blood.

In some hospitals, O Rhesus Negative blood is a very rare commodity. In these circumstances, and when there is critical hypovolaemia, O Rhesus Positive blood may be given, but this is not desirable in young women whose Rhesus status is unknown.

[1]Barnes A. Transfusions of universal donor and uncrossmatched blood. *Bibl Haematologica* 1980; **46**: 132.

The stabbed stay stabbed until they reach theatre

The reason

An impaling object may tamponade a blood vessel it has injured. If the object is removed outside the operating theatre, the resultant haemorrhage may be uncontrollable.

A knife is a sharp instrument and can cause as much damage on the way out from cutting as on the way in. Therefore explore the wound under anaesthetic and control any major blood vessel (slings and/or clamps) before removing the impaling object.

The exceptions

Small impaling objects in anatomically non-vital tissues may be removed with caution in the emergency department.

An injury above and below the abdomen implies an injury IN the abdomen

The reason

The abdomen has little bony protection and its contents are vulnerable. For victims of blunt trauma, especially a motor vehicle accident where there has been diffuse blunt impact,* there should be a high index of suspicion for occult abdominal injury if there are obvious injuries above and below the abdomen.

* Imagine a pedestrian being hit by a bus.

The exceptions

Penetrating trauma above and below the abdomen does not necessarily indicate injury to the abdomen, although a gunshot wound with an entry in the thigh and exit in the chest **must** have traversed the abdomen, and a stab wound of the chest can involve the abdomen if the blade was long enough and directed caudally (see Rule 23).

The exception in blunt trauma is the patient hit by a giant flying horseshoe.

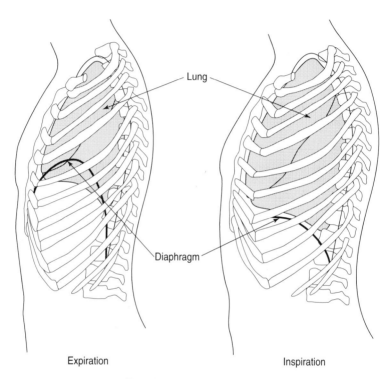

Lung

Diaphragm

Expiration

Inspiration

Excursion of the diaphragm during
inspiration and expiration

On expiration the diaphragm may rise to the level of the fourth intercostal space
anteriorly.

A penetrating wound below the nipple involves the abdomen

The reason

On expiration the diaphragm will rise anteriorly to approximately the level of the nipple in men. A penetrating wound at or below this level should be presumed to involve the chest **and** abdominal cavities.

To get into the abdomen from the chest, a penetrating object must pass through the diaphragm. Even in the absence of intra-abdominal visceral injury there may be immediate or delayed rupture of the diaphragm.

To exclude diaphragmatic involvement, a laparoscopy or thoracoscopy would be the investigation of choice. Less satisfactorily, or when abdominal visceral involvement is sought, a *diagnostic peritoneal lavage* (DPL) can be performed in an adult (see Rule 42). If the DPL is negative the patient can be observed and re-examined at intervals; if it is positive an operation is required. Free blood in the abdomen of a child is not necessarily an indication for an operation, as some visceral injuries can be treated conservatively. A CT scan will define the injury and may allow a conservative approach.

The exceptions

If the patient was stabbed or shot during inspiration, then the injuries may be confined to the chest.

The nipple is not a reliable surface marker in women.

The false negative rate for diagnostic peritoneal lavage with an isolated rupture of the diaphragm is 12–40% for penetrating trauma (14–36% for blunt trauma). The threshold for operative intervention is therefore reduced to when the red blood cell count is greater than $5 \times 10^6/l$ in the peritoneal lavage fluid.[1]

[1]Moore EE, Marx JA. Penetrating abdominal wounds. Rationale for exploratory laparotomy. *JAMA* 1985; **253**: 2705.

Examination of the abdomen is as reliable as flipping a coin

The reason

The absence of clinical symptoms and signs of peritonism does not reliably exclude free intra-abdominal blood following trauma. In fact, symptoms and signs may be absent in up to 40% of patients.[1] Furthermore, signs may be masked in a patient who is unconscious, intoxicated, or who has a high spinal cord injury with loss of abdominal sensation.

In those without symptoms and signs a high index of suspicion must be maintained, together with close observation of the pulse, blood pressure, and respiratory rate. If there is doubt then further investigations should be performed (diagnostic peritoneal lavage or CT of the abdomen).

The exceptions

If there are abdominal signs and the patient is haemodynamically unstable, then surgery is mandatory. Investigations impose a delay in management and are contraindicated.

[1]Rossoff L, Cohen JL, Telfer N, *et al.* Injuries of the spleen. *Surg Clin North Am* 1972; **52**: 667.

Neurogenic shock is hypovolaemic shock until proved otherwise

The reason

Neurogenic shock describes the loss of vascular tone when the sympathetic nervous system is interrupted in a high spinal cord injury. The result is peripheral venous pooling and hypotension.

Hypovolaemic shock is much more common than neurogenic shock, and hypovolaemia may coexist with a spinal cord injury. It is much safer to assume that the shock is a result of hypovolaemia and to start fluid resuscitation while looking for the cause. If you treat neurogenic shock as hypovolaemia you are unlikely to harm the patient, but the converse is not true.

This table may help you to differentiate between hypovolaemic shock and neurogenic shock.

	Hypovolaemic shock	*Neurogenic shock*
Pulse rate	↑	→/↓
Pulse pressure	↓	↑
Skin	Clammy, pale, cold	Dry, flushed, warm
Systolic BP	→/↓	→/↓
Urine output	↓	↓

The exceptions

Once hypovolaemic shock has been excluded, specific treatments for neurogenic shock include atropine for bradycardia and vasopressors (ephedrine and phenylephrine) for low vascular tone.

Neurogenic shock should be differentiated from spinal shock, which is a temporary loss of tone and spinal reflexes below the level of the injury.

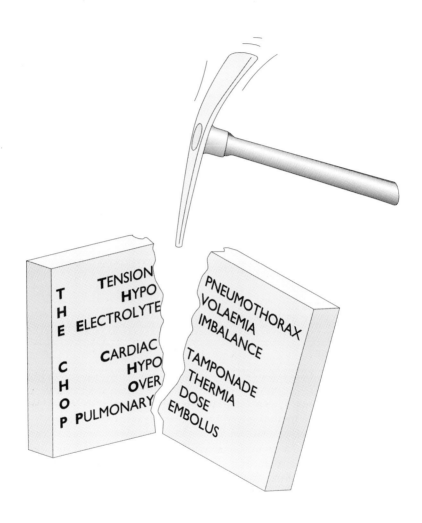

Think of the EMD causes or your patient is for THE CHOP.

Think of the EMD causes or your patient is for THE CHOP

The reason

Electromechanical dissociation (EMD) is co-ordinated electrical activity without a pulse. It is one of the four primary cardiac arrest rhythms (ventricular fibrillation, pulseless ventricular tachycardia, asystole, and EMD). Some causes of EMD will be more common following a traumatic than a "medical" cardiac arrest, and these include tension pneumothorax, hypovolaemia, and cardiac tamponade. But do not forget that the other components of THE CHOP may occur in trauma: electrolyte imbalance following massive transfusion; hypothermia associated with the injury; the drugged patient involved in an accident; and a pulmonary embolus following surgery and bed rest (or air embolus in penetrating chest injury).

T   Tension pneumothorax
H   Hypovolaemia
E   Electrolyte imbalance

C   Cardiac tamponade
H   Hypothermia
O   Overdose
P   Pulmonary embolus

The exceptions

The European Resuscitation Council guidelines (1992) for EMD are to start basic life support, consider treatable causes, intubate and obtain intravenous access, give adrenaline 1 mg intravenously and repeat this twice, then consider 5 mg adrenaline intravenously.

It is very important to treat the underlying causes of EMD, but basic life support must be maintained and repeated adrenaline should not be forgotten. Therefore, think of one or two causes and treat them on each loop of the EMD protocol (for example think of hypovolaemia and tension pneumothorax on the first loop; think of cardiac tamponade and hypothermia on the second loop).

> *Think of the causes to begin,*
> *And treat them if you want to win.*
> *Then tube, IV, adrenaline,*
> *Cycles* one to five by ten,*
> *If no improvement round again.*

* 1 × ventilation to 5 × chest compressions.

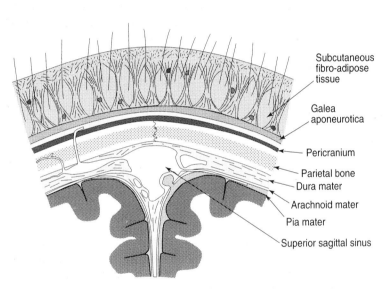

Subcutaneous fibro-adipose tissue

Galea aponeurotica

Pericranium

Parietal bone

Dura mater

Arachnoid mater

Pia mater

Superior sagittal sinus

A coronal section showing the anatomical layers of the scalp and skull.

Head injury alone does not cause hypotension

The reason

The brain is contained within a rigid box and this box can only accommodate a small intracranial haemorrhage, insufficient to produce hypotension.

The initial compensatory mechanisms for an expanding intracranial haematoma are for blood and CSF to be squeezed out of the brain. This helps to maintain a near normal intracranial pressure (ICP). However, when these compensatory mechanisms fail, a further small rise in volume can lead to a large increase in ICP.

As little as 50–100 ml of blood may overwhelm the compensatory mechanisms. At this time the brain will herniate through the tentorium cerebelli (uncus of the temporal lobe presses against the third nerve causing ipsilateral pupil dilatation) and the foramen magnum ("coning": death follows compression of the respiratory and cardiovascular centres in the brainstem).

As intracranial pressure rises a combination of *hypertension* and bradycardia may be seen, known as the Cushing response.

The exceptions

Infants have a small circulating blood volume and a semi-rigid box enclosing the brain. The skull may expand because fontanelles can bulge and sutures can be stretched. Infants can therefore become shocked as a result of intracranial blood loss.

The scalp has a rich blood supply and significant haemorrhage can occur from a scalp laceration in children or adults. Additionally, a haemorrhage between the galea and the skull (a cephalhaematoma) in small infants may be large enough to produce signs of hypovolaemia.

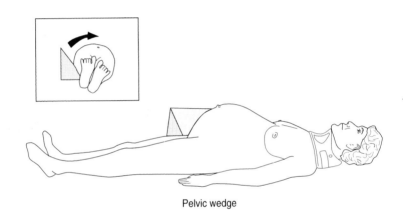

Pelvic wedge

Resuscitate the mother and the baby will look after itself.

Resuscitate the mother and the baby will look after itself

The reason

With trauma in pregnancy, the priority is to resuscitate the mother. If the mother is adequately oxygenated and perfused, then so will be the foetus.

In the supine position, the gravid uterus may compress the inferior vena cava and greatly reduce the venous return to the heart. This produces a *supine hypotension syndrome*, where both the maternal and foetal circulation is impaired. It is therefore important, as part of the resuscitation of "circulation", to place a pelvic wedge under the RIGHT hip to displace the uterus from the inferior vena cava. If there is a strong suspicion of thoracolumbar spinal injury and concern about placing the wedge, then the uterus can be displaced manually.

The exceptions

Emergency delivery of the baby may still be required as soon as possible, especially if resuscitative attempts directed towards the mother are failing.

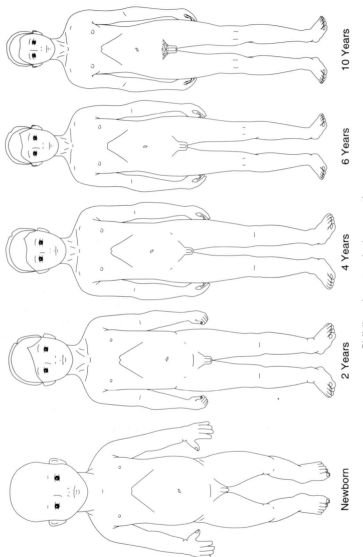

Childhood anatomical proportions.

Newborn 2 Years 4 Years 6 Years 10 Years

Children are not small adults

The reason

There are important anatomical and physiological differences in children (for example the epiglottis is floppy and leaf-like in a small child; the blood volume is ~80 ml/kg in children and ~70 ml/kg in adults) which mean you cannot simply use smaller versions of the same adult equipment or a proportionally reduced dose of a particular drug.

Instead, there are paediatric formulae to estimate weight, the appropriate diameter and length of an endotracheal tube, and systolic blood pressure.

- Weight (kg)* $= [\text{age (years)} + 4] \times 2$
- Endotracheal tube
  internal diameter (mm) $= [\text{age (years)} \div 4] + 4$
- Systolic blood pressure $= 80 + [\text{age (years)} \times 2]$

* Accurate from age 1–10 years.

Drug doses for children are expressed in dose per kilogram. But you do not have to remember all of these; normal values for children and the doses of important resuscitation drugs are contained on commercial paediatric resuscitation charts (such as the *Revised Oakley Paediatric Resuscitation Chart*[1] or the *Broselow Tape*).

The exceptions

Despite the differences in anatomy and physiology, the principles of trauma resuscitation remain the same for children and adults, namely:

Airway
Breathing
Circulation.

[1] Oakley P, Phillips B, Molyneux E, Mackway-Jones K. Paediatric resuscitation. Updated standard reference chart. *BMJ* 1993; **306**: 1096–8.

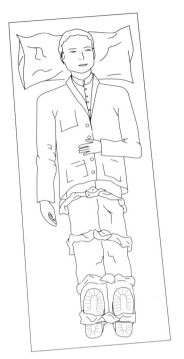

Simple splintage for a fractured femur.

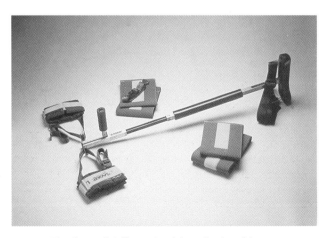

Traction splint (Sager type) for a fractured femur.

Limb splintage is part of resuscitation

The reason

Limb splintage relieves pain and may reduce blood loss. Pain releases catecholamines which cause peripheral vasoconstriction, and this may further reduce the oxygen delivery to an injured periphery. Pain also produces a tachycardia which increases myocardial oxygen demand: this may be unfavourable in existing myocardial disease or after blunt myocardial trauma.

Blood loss from a fractured femur can be further reduced by a *traction splint*. The effect is mechanical by changing the shape of the swollen thigh from a sphere to an ovoid which holds less fluid. The Thomas Splint (Hugh Owen Thomas) was the first traction splint, and when used extensively in the First World War it reduced the mortality of an open fractured femur from 80% to 20%. Modern traction splints (Hare Splint, Donway Splint) use the same principle of traction at the ankle and counter-traction at the ischial tuberosity, except the Sager Splint which exerts counter-traction against the symphysis pubis.

A particularly valuable feature of the Sager Splint is that it can immobilise bilateral femur fractures while still allowing the patient to fit on the ambulance cot or resuscitation trolley.

The exceptions

The desire to splint a bleeding, fractured limb should not distract the clinician from their most important priorities: airway and breathing first!

Traction on a supracondylar fracture of the femur may cause the distal fragment to tilt posteriorly and impinge on the popliteal vessels. Traction should be applied with caution in this circumstance.

It is important to ensure that displaced fractures and dislocated joints are anatomically realigned as soon as possible and not just splinted. Pressure and traction forces will be exerted on adjacent blood vessels, nerves, and ligaments. The blood supply to the skin, for example, may be compromised and pressure necrosis can develop rapidly (common with a fracture-dislocation of the ankle).

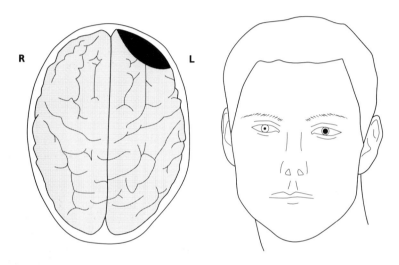

Pupil dilated same side as injury

Assessment of pupils.

The Glasgow Coma Scale does not measure prognosis

The reason

The Glasgow Coma Scale (GCS) is a measure of brain function at the time the test is performed. It is not an indicator of prognosis. The GCS is a summative assessment of the best motor, and eye-opening responses, with a maximum score of 15 and a minimum score of 3. If there is a different response in opposite limbs then the best response is recorded.

Motor response	Verbal response	Eye opening
6 Obeys commands	5 Orientated	4 Spontaneous
5 Localises pain	4 Confused	3 To voice
4 Withdraws from pain	3 Inappropriate words	2 To pain
3 Abnormal flexion	2 Groans	1 None
2 Extension to pain	1 None	
1 None		

In general, a GCS of <9 indicates a severe head injury, a GCS between 9 and 12 indicates a moderate head injury, and a GCS >12 suggests a mild head injury. However this can be misleading, since the GCS can be reduced to as low as 3 in a hypoxic patient without a significant head injury, and a patient developing a potentially lethal extradural haemorrhage may be fully alert with a GCS of 15 during the "lucid interval". It is much more important to record the trend in GCS over time and to be wary of changes in the level of response. If the GCS falls by 2 points or more, this is a significant deterioration.

The neurological examination in trauma would not be complete without an assessment of pupils and a search for lateralising signs (unilateral weakness or altered sensation).

The exceptions

The GCS is used as an outcome measure when incorporated into one of the physiological scoring systems, such as the Trauma Score, Revised Trauma Score, or the Triage Revised Trauma Score.[1]

---

[1]Yates DW. Scoring systems. In: Skinner D, Driscoll P, Earlam R. *ABC of Major Trauma*, 2nd edn. London: BMJ Publishing Group, 1996.

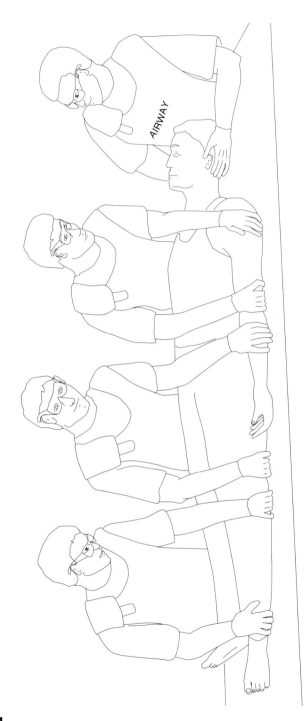

The log roll.
The doctor or nurse holding the head will give the orders controlling the roll.

A patient has a front and a back, two sides, a top and a bottom

The reason

If injuries are not to be missed each patient must be completely exposed and rolled in a controlled manner on to their side to look at the back (the so-called *log roll*). Missed wounds on the back can be a cause of fatal exsanguination. The index of suspicion should be particularly high with penetrating trauma. Do not assume the patient has a single frontal stab wound. If you can only see one bullet wound, are you missing the exit (or entrance) wound on the back?

The exceptions

Complete exposure has to be considered in the context of the patient's environment, which is particularly true outside hospital. Additionally, in the pre-hospital phase, time would not permit complete exposure and examination and the emphasis is on ABC priorities.

Once in hospital you need to see all of the patient, but not necessarily all at the same time. Children have a larger surface area to volume ratio than adults and will cool very quickly, especially if they are wet and immobile through injury or coma. Active measures should be taken to protect the patient from hypothermia (see Rule 35).

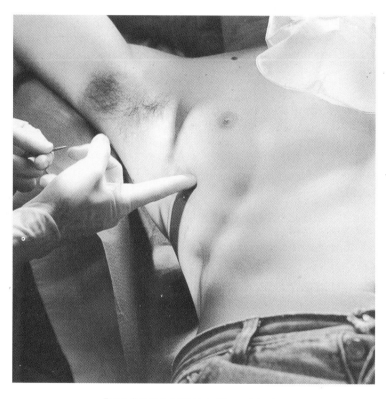

Put a finger in before putting a tube in.

Put a finger in before putting a tube in

The reason

After blunt dissection through the chest wall, a 360° finger sweep should be performed before inserting a chest drain. This will exclude a pleural adhesion (in which case an alternative site for the drain should be sought) or intrathoracic abdominal contents (in which case the drain must be inserted since a pneumothorax has now been produced, but the patient is not anticipated to improve without surgery to repair the diaphragm).

A rectal examination is required before inserting a urinary catheter in men to identify the possibility of urethral injury, which is suggested by a high-riding prostate. Other signs will be perineal or scrotal bruising, an inability to pass urine, and blood at the meatus. The rectal examination is also useful to exclude blood in the bowel from bowel injury and check sphincter tone, which may be absent in spinal cord injury.

The little finger of the patient can be used as a rough guide, particularly in children, to estimate the correct internal diameter of the endotracheal tube.

The exceptions

If the integrity of the urethra has been confirmed by urethrography, a catheter may be passed. A urethrogram is performed by introducing a soft catheter tip into the meatus and then injecting 15–20 ml of water-soluble contrast. Any extravasation indicates a rupture, and complete rupture is suggested by a failure of contrast to enter the bladder. If urethral rupture is diagnosed, a suprapubic catheter should be passed and the opinion of a urologist sought.

The technique of diagnostic peritoneal lavage, although best performed as an open procedure, does not generally require a finger to be inserted into the abdominal cavity.

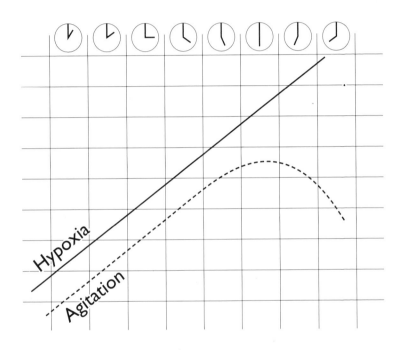

The agitated patient will calm down whilst deteriorating.

The agitated patient will calm down whilst deteriorating

The reason

Moderate hypoxia will lead to disorientation, aggression, and a tendency to be abusive to the attending medical staff. If nothing is done to improve oxygenation, the patient's cerebral function will deteriorate and he or she will drift into unconsciousness. This is a pre-terminal event, but may be misinterpreted as an improvement by those struggling to control an individual who has been fighting every attempt at assessment and treatment.

It may be necessary to anaesthetise, paralyse and ventilate an agitated patient in order to secure an airway and maintain adequate respiration. Causes of agitation other than hypoxia can then be investigated in a controlled fashion.

The exceptions

Agitation is common in trauma patients, particularly as a result of anxiety and pain. It is important to reassure the patient and to explain any procedure during the resuscitation to ensure maximum co-operation.

The causes of agitation to consider in a trauma victim are:

- Hypoxia (obstructed airway, chest injury, hypovolaemia)
- Cerebral irritation (cerebral oedema, intracranial haemorrhage)
- Pain
- Anxiety
- Full bladder
- Alcohol and other substance abuse

Sedating an agitated patient to allow the airway and ventilation to be controlled is acceptable. But sedation alone does not treat the cause of agitation, which must be actively sought and managed.

Rule 35

You are not dead until you are death warmed up

The reason

Hypothermia is a core temperature of <35°C (mild 32–35°C, moderate 30–32°C, severe <30°C). Asystole will appear at very low temperatures (18–20°C), and it may be inappropriate to pronounce death without first attempting to re-warm the body as the asystole can be reversible. Ventricular fibrillation may not respond to DC shocks until the core temperature is >30°C. Methods of **reversing** hypothermia are *passive* and *active*.

Passive	Warm blankets Warm-air duvet
Active	Warm intravenous fluids Warm intragastric, intracystic, and intraperitoneal fluid lavage Thoracic heat cradle

Hypothermia is commonly seen in patients with major trauma (where *major trauma* is defined as an Injury Severity Score* of ⩾16), being found in 21% of these patients.[1] It is therefore very important to **prevent** hypothermia.

- Remove wet clothing/sheets and dry the patient.
- Warm any intravenous fluids that are needed.[†]
- Cover with blankets when not examining the patient or performing a procedure.
- Use an overhead heater or air-heated duvet (Bear-hugger™, Warm-Touch™).

* The Injury Severity Score is an anatomical scoring system that is a summative score of the most serious injuries in up to three of six body regions.
† Blood should be warmed to body temperature (a Level 1 blood warmer is much more efficient than a coil warmer); colloid and crystalloid should be stored in a warm cabinet at body temperature.

The exceptions

Re-warming is inappropriate when there is rigor mortis or a cause of death that is clearly incompatible with resuscitation (such as decapitation).

[1]Gunning K, Sugrue M, Sloan D, Deane S. Hypothermia and severe trauma. *Aust NZ J Surg* 1995; **65**: 80–2.

The golden rule is golden fluid in the golden hour

The reason

A urine output of over 50 ml/hour in an adult confirms adequate fluid resuscitation. If the urine output is less than 30 ml/hour following injury, there should be a strong suspicion of significant uncorrected hypovolaemia.

In a child, aim to achieve at least 2 ml/kg/hour of urine; less than 1 ml/kg/hour should be considered to represent oliguria.

In burns resuscitation it is common to use a fluid resuscitation formula.

- Parkland formula (crystalloid)
  weight (kg) × % burn × 4 = ml crystalloid per 24 hours (half in first 8 hours)
- Muir and Barclay formula (colloid)
  [weight (kg) × % burn] ÷ 2 = ml colloid per unit time*

* Units of time are 4 hr, 4 hr, 4 hr, 6 hr, 6 hr, 12 hr.

These resuscitation formulae are just a guide and it is important to adjust the fluids according to the urine output. In children it is more accurate to use a Burns Calculator.[1]

The exceptions

A diuresis may be induced by hypothermia and may produce hypovolaemia. This "cold diuresis" may lead to a false sense of security during the resuscitation of a hypothermic patient and is a result of a decreased reabsorption of sodium and water in the kidneys.[2]

[1]Milner S, Hodgetts T, Rylah A. The Burns Calculator: a simple proposed guide for fluid replacement. *Lancet* 1993; **342**: 1089–91.
[2]Fischer R, Souba W, Ford E. Temperature-associated injuries and syndromes. In: Moore E, Mattox K, Feliciano D. *Trauma.* Connecticut: Appleton and Lange, 1991.

Rule 37

It doesn't hurt to give analgesia

The reason

There is no excuse for leaving a patient in pain. Pain results in the release of catecholamines which cause peripheral and splanchnic vasoconstriction. Since hypovolaemia produces the same catecholamine response, pain will exacerbate the physiological response to hypovolaemic shock.

Pain relief can be achieved by:

- Reassurance
- Splintage
- Nitrous oxide (50 : 50 mixture with oxygen, as Entonox or Nitronox)
- Opiates, for example morphine, diamorphine (given intravenously)
- Other parenteral drugs, for example ketamine
- Local anaesthesia, for example femoral nerve block

Opiates must be given intravenously as intramuscular absorption is unreliable when peripheral perfusion is reduced. Ketamine is a powerful analgesic drug at 0·5–1·0 mg/kg IV, and at 2 mg/kg it is an anaesthetic agent. Beware of hypersalivation and emergence delirium with the higher dose. Possibility of the latter can be reduced by a small concomitant dose of benzodiazepine. A femoral nerve block can give **complete** pain relief for a mid-shaft fracture of the femur, but it is unreliable with femoral neck and supracondylar fractures.

The exceptions

Traditionally, it has been taught not to give opiates with a chest injury as they may depress respiration. This is unlikely if they are given in small aliquots, and ventilation may be improved by relieving the chest pain. Opiates have also been maligned in head injury as they may reduce the level of response and alter pupillary signs, so making assessment of the neurological status difficult. Again, if small aliquots are given these are not significant concerns.

Nitrous oxide is contraindicated in chest injury where pneumothorax is present or suspected: a pneumothorax may rapidly tension when the nitrous oxide diffuses into it. Nitrous oxide is also contraindicated with decompression sickness ("the bends" or caisson disease) and when the patient is unable to co-operate and self-administer the drug.

The team leader is always right

The reason

For a trauma team to run effectively, there must be an identifiable leader who will make the key clinical decisions. Members of the team must respect this authority and be prepared to carry out the leader's instructions.

The exceptions

A good team leader will support and encourage the team and will allow their instructions to be questioned. The team leader cannot always be right, but after discussion the leader **must** make the final decision.

If in doubt, call the trauma team

The reason

You may be afraid of your ability to manage a seriously injured patient. This is natural. When you stop being afraid of your abilities and become complacent, this is the time to worry. But you should never be afraid to ask for help.

In many hospitals the trauma team will be called according to established criteria, based on the history of the incident, the anatomical injury and the abnormal vital signs.

- History
  - Fall >6 metres
  - Pedestrian or cyclist hit by a car
  - Other occupant killed
  - Ejected from vehicle
- Injuries
  - >1 long bone fractured (radius and ulna on the same side count as 1)
  - >1 anatomical area injured
  - Penetrating injury to the torso or head
  - >15% burns (>10% in child)
  - Traumatic amputation or crush injury
- Vital signs
  - Respiratory rate >29/minute
  - Pulse rate >130 or <50/minute
  - Systolic BP <90 mm Hg
  - Glasgow Coma Scale <13

The exceptions

When the trauma team is activated on mechanism of injury alone (the history), there will be a significant proportion of cases where no serious pathology is found. However, this is the price to pay for not missing those with serious occult injury (see Rule 3).

Investigation and definitive care

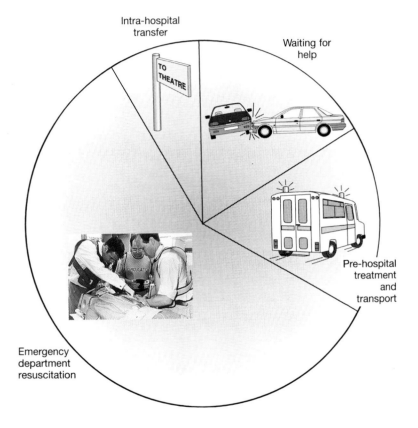

Intra-hospital transfer

Waiting for help

Pre-hospital treatment and transport

Emergency department resuscitation

The golden hour.

The golden hour belongs to the patient

The reason

The *golden hour* is the "ideal" time from injury to definitive treatment in the operating theatre. This must include the time to mobilise the emergency services, to treat the patient at the scene, to transport the patient to hospital and to resuscitate within the emergency department.

The golden hour does not therefore belong to the emergency services at the scene, nor does the clock start on arrival at hospital – it is already ticking.

It may be appropriate to think in terms of a *platinum ten minutes* to stabilise the patient at the scene, and certainly for the ambulance service personnel to ask themselves every ten minutes the question, "Why am I still here?"

The exceptions

In some situations the golden hour will slip by unavoidably. These are:

- Entrapment, for example at a road traffic accident
- Difficult or remote environment for rescue (e.g. cliffs)

In patients with penetrating trauma, the decision to operate is usually obvious. With multi-system blunt trauma it is often necessary to perform investigations before a decision to operate is made, for example a CT scan of the brain or a diagnostic peritoneal lavage. These investigations will encroach on the golden hour.

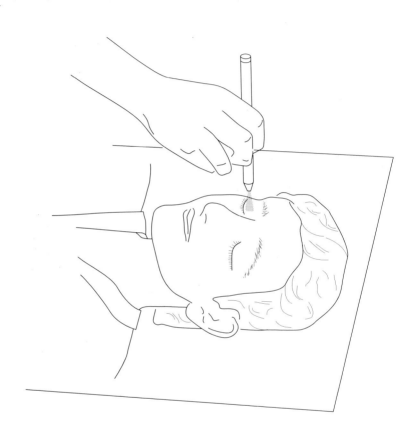

You can assess vision with the eyes closed.

You can assess vision with the eyes closed

The reason

Following facial injury the periorbital tissues can swell rapidly, making assessment of the eyes very difficult.

Gross optic nerve function can be assessed through a swollen lid by asking a conscious patient if the light from a pen-torch held against the lid can be seen.

The exceptions

The following cannot be assessed through a closed lid:

- Pupillary reaction to light
- Eye movements
- Structural intraorbital injury
- Visual acuity

If the eyes are open, visual acuity should be tested in the resuscitation room, but it will not be possible to formally assess this using a Snellen chart, unless an appropriately scaled chart is placed on the ceiling above the head end of the trolley. Instead, it is acceptable to test the ability to read print on a chart or drug carton.

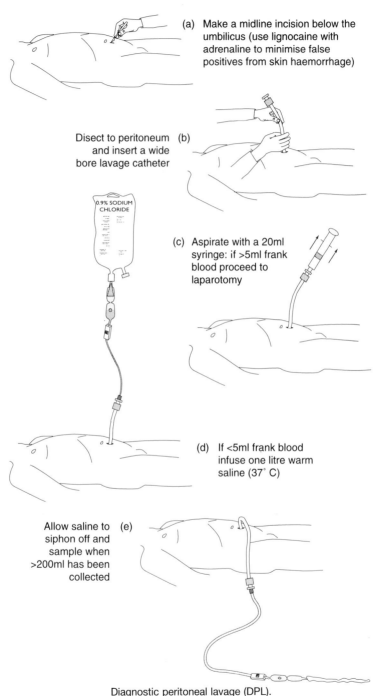

(a) Make a midline incision below the umbilicus (use lignocaine with adrenaline to minimise false positives from skin haemorrhage)

Disect to peritoneum (b) and insert a wide bore lavage catheter

(c) Aspirate with a 20ml syringe: if >5ml frank blood proceed to laparotomy

0.9% SODIUM CHLORIDE

(d) If <5ml frank blood infuse one litre warm saline (37° C)

Allow saline to (e) siphon off and sample when >200ml has been collected

Diagnostic peritoneal lavage (DPL).

You may read the newspaper, but you cannot read the DPL

The reason

It has been stated that if newsprint is legible through the fluid in the drainage bag from a diagnostic peritoneal lavage (DPL) then the test is negative. This method is unscientific and has no place in the objective assessment and management of potential intra-abdominal injury.

When performed and interpreted correctly, the diagnostic peritoneal lavage is a sensitive, although non-specific, investigation which can detect as little as 20 ml of free blood in the peritoneal cavity. It may also be used to detect perforation of the small or large bowel.

A sample of the drained effluent should be sent to the laboratory for analysis of red blood cell count, white blood cell count, alkaline phosphatase (to detect occult bowel injury)[1] and Gram's stain. Arrangements for urgent processing should be made.

Finding	Interpretation	Action
$>1 \times 10^8$ rbc/l	Positive	Laparotomy
$0.5–1 \times 10^8$ rbc/l	Equivocal	Reassess, investigate further
$<0.5 \times 10^8$ rbc/l	Negative	Observe (chance of missed injury 1–2%)
$>5 \times 10^5$ wbc/l	Positive	Laparotomy
Bacteria or particulate matter	Equivocal	Reassess, investigate further
Faeces	Positive	Laparotomy
Alkaline phosphatase >10 U/l	Positive	Laparotomy (probable small bowel injury)

The exceptions

Aspiration of frank blood on insertion of the DPL catheter is a positive result and requires a laparotomy to be performed in an adult. As some intra-abdominal injuries in children may be managed conservatively, it is important to quantify the structural damage. A CT scan would often be preferred to a DPL in children.

[1] Jaffin J, Ochsner M, Cole F, et al. Alkaline phosphatase levels in diagnostic peritoneal lavage fluid as a predictor of hollow visceral injury. *Journal of Trauma* 1993; **34(6)**: 829–33.

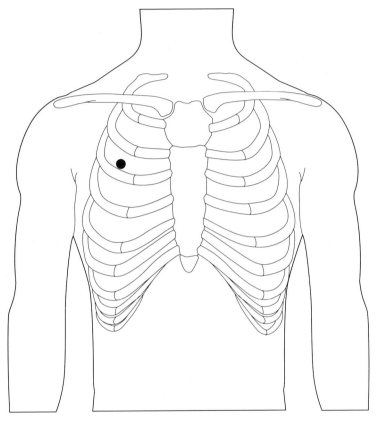

● Second intercostal space, mid-clavicular line

Surface markings for needle thoracocentesis. To find the second intercostal space, place your finger at the top of the sternum and move down until you feel a ridge (sternal angle). Now move laterally on to the second rib as far as the mid-clavicular line. Go below the second rib into the second intercostal space.

A tension pneumothorax cannot be diagnosed on a chest x-ray

The reason

A tension pneumothorax is an immediately life-threatening emergency. It is a clinical diagnosis and it is inappropriate to wait for a chest x-ray to confirm the diagnosis. If you diagnose it, you must treat it – immediately!

	Tension pneumothorax
Symptoms	*Signs*
Respiratory distress	Increased respiratory rate
	Tachycardia and hypotension
	Cyanosis
	Hyperinflated, resonant chest
	Absent breath sounds
	Tracheal deviation (away from affected side)
	Distended neck veins
	Confusion, extending to coma

The treatment of tension pneumothorax is needle decompression via a large-bore cannula in the second intercostal space, mid-clavicular line. This relieves the tension but there will still be a complete pneumothorax. A chest drain is required.

The exceptions

There are no exceptions to this rule, but it is frightening how often a chest x-ray that shows a tension pneumothorax will be seen.

Rule 44

A supine chest x-ray may be worse than no chest x-ray at all

The reason

A chest x-ray in the trauma resuscitation room is looking for:

- Pneumothorax
- Haemothorax
- Widened mediastinum
- Air under the diaphragm (perforated hollow viscus)

The presence of any of these will influence the immediate management of the patient, but all of them can easily be missed on a supine chest x-ray.

When possible, the patient should be sat up at the earliest opportunity for an erect chest x-ray. Following blunt trauma, a supine chest x-ray will still be performed as one of the primary survey x-rays until the spine has been cleared clinically and radiographically – but consider tilting the complete bed by 20° head up. This may help you see a haemothorax (fluid level, rather than generalised increase in density of hemithorax), a small pneumothorax (at the apex), and air under the diaphragm (when supine, free air will be found at the centre of the abdomen and will be missed on the chest film).

In the case of a widened mediastinum on a supine film, which implies a possible contained aortic disruption, an erect chest x-ray could save the patient from the unnecessarily high dose of radiation of a CT scan or dangerous arch aortography. But do remember that the preferred investigation for a widened mediastinum (>8 cm in adults) is an arch aortogram, as both CT and MRI have been shown to be less sensitive.[1]

The exceptions

There is no reason to perform a supine chest x-ray following penetrating trauma except when there is a clinical suspicion of spinal involvement or the patient is profoundly hypotensive. Primary survey chest x-rays in these cases should be erect/semi-erect.

[1]Miller F, Richardson J, Thomas H. Role of CT scanning in the diagnosis of major arterial injury after blunt thoracic trauma. *Surgery* 1989; **106**: 596.

Investigation must never impede resuscitation

The reason

Investigations are available to:

- Clarify equivocal signs, for example diagnostic peritoneal lavage (DPL)
- Confirm clinical suspicions, for example CT brain scan
- Plan management, for example x-ray long bones

It is important that these investigations do not interfere with resuscitation along ABC lines. If a patient clinically has an abdomen distended with blood, a laparotomy is required, not a DPL. Equally, a life-saving operation for intra-abdominal haemorrhage takes precedence over a CT scan of the spine for suspected spinal injury. The patient will die immediately from blood loss, but will not (in general) die immediately in hospital from a spinal injury.

The exceptions

Investigations are also available to rule out clinically undetected injury, for example primary survey x-rays. The primary survey x-rays are part of the resuscitation, as the following serious injuries can easily be missed clinically:

Chest	pneumothorax or haemothorax
	contained aortic rupture
Pelvis	stable pelvic fracture
Cervical spine	fracture or dislocation

Obtaining blood for cross-match is part of the trauma resuscitation and is best done immediately after insertion of an intravenous cannula. A blood glucose estimation (capillary test is enough initially, for example BM-stix or Glucostix) should be considered part of the resuscitation in children, as hypoglycaemia is a common sequela of childhood illness or injury.

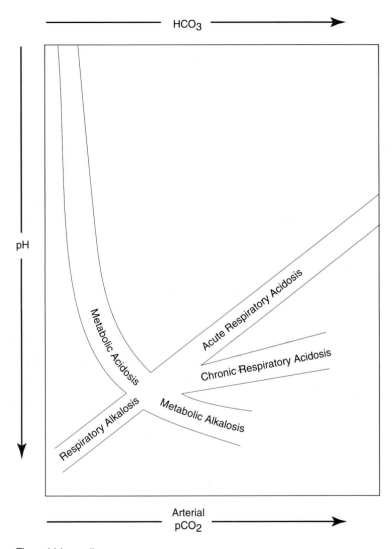

The acid-base diagram.

Serial blood gases are the signposts on the road to resuscitation

The reason

Shock is present when there is inadequate organ perfusion and tissue oxygenation, leading to anaerobic respiration and lactic acidosis. Lactic acidosis can be quantified as the *base excess*, which can be measured from an arterial sample of blood.

If resuscitation of a shocked patient is effective, tissue perfusion will improve, the lactate will be cleared and the base excess will move towards normal. If it is inadequate, lactate will accumulate further and the base excess will continue to deteriorate.

Serial arterial blood gas estimations should be performed on every severely injured patient in hospital, and should be repeated at regular intervals during the resuscitation.

The exceptions

If there is a clear clinical indication to pass an endotracheal tube, do not wait for blood gas results before deciding to intubate.

In trauma cardiac arrest, there is a reduced volume of CO_2 delivered to the alveoli for clearance. A *paradoxical respiratory alkalosis* can be seen when there is arterial hypocarbia, despite the persistent venous acidosis due to the high venous concentrations of CO_2 and lactic acid. Following cardiac arrest, a central venous sample should be used to determine the patient's pH, while an arterial sample will determine whether the patient is being adequately oxygenated.[1]

[1]Advanced Life Support Group. *Advanced Cardiac Life Support.* London: Chapman & Hall, 1993.

77

The radiology department is a dangerous place

The reason

It is often tempting to send a patient to the radiology department for diagnostic plain films or computed tomography (CT) scan, but these departments are poorly equipped to deal with a patient who suddenly deteriorates.

First think if the investigation is essential to the immediate management of the patient, or whether it can be performed adequately on portable equipment in the emergency department. Portable films should also be kept to a minimum, and are usually restricted to a series of three films (lateral cervical spine, chest, and pelvis) to limit the exposure to radiation of the patient and emergency department staff, which is greater with portable equipment. However, quickly taken portable films of long-bone fractures may help the orthopaedic surgeons to plan surgery that is to run concurrently with or immediately after life-saving surgery to the chest, abdomen, or head. Such films should not delay the transfer of a patient to theatre for life-saving procedures.

The exceptions

CT is useful in diagnosing a range of occult traumatic injuries and will help the clinician to plan the best course of treatment. It has revolutionised the approach to traumatic head injury. Adequate equipment and appropriately trained staff **must** accompany any seriously injured patient who is being moved to the CT scanner or any other department. Remember that during radiation exposure in the CT scanner the patient is unattended and difficult to monitor. It is therefore safer to secure the airway of an obtunded trauma patient in the controlled environment of the emergency department before moving to the CT scanner.

Magnetic resonance imaging (MRI) is inappropriate in acute multi-system trauma. Metal components of resuscitation equipment cannot enter the scanner, which is also extremely claustraphobic with restricted patient access.

Alternatives to radiology should be considered. In an adult, diagnostic peritoneal lavage is a rapid and sensitive tool for detecting free intraperitoneal blood and deciding the need for laparotomy. Portable ultrasound can also be used for children and adults in the emergency department to detect intra-abdominal free fluid and solid organ disruption.

Patients are transferred, not their injuries or investigations

The reason

All patients are people. If we forget this we are simply technicians, not clinicians.

So remember to say, *"This is Mr Smith. He is 40 and has a ruptured spleen"*, rather than, *"This is the 40-year-old ruptured spleen"*.

Also, consider that relatives may be within earshot of the resuscitation room or in the resuscitation room (particularly in the case of paediatric trauma). What you say is often remembered.

The exceptions

The expression, *"This is the kidney for theatre."* may be used to refer to the donor organ!

Rule 49

Never believe a transferring hospital

The reason

When a patient is transferred from one hospital to another the receiving hospital must perform a complete reassessment. Injuries may have been missed by the initial hospital, or the patient may have deteriorated in transit. The trauma team should be activated to assess an inter-hospital transfer. A particular problem is the patient with multi-system trauma referred to a second hospital for a CT brain scan who goes straight to the CT scanner and bypasses the emergency department. Remember that the radiology department is a dangerous place (see Rule 47).

Sick patients transfer badly. Monitoring is less accurate when moving, and treatment is restricted. Always ensure that the airway, breathing, and circulation are stable before transfer. Elective intubation should be considered if any problems with the airway or ventilation are anticipated. It is relatively easy to do this in the controlled environment of the emergency department, but very difficult to do in an ambulance when the patient suddenly deteriorates. The patient must have an appropriately qualified escort. In the case of inter-hospital transfer of a seriously injured patient, this would usually be a doctor with anaesthetic and trauma resuscitation skills.

When accepting a trauma patient from another hospital, it is important to remember that the referring hospital may not deal with major trauma on a regular basis. Give helpful advice and do not be patronising. More importantly, give the referring hospital feedback so that the staff involved regard the episode positively and continue to learn.

The exceptions

If a retrieval team has gone from the receiving hospital to collect the patient, then there is a continuity of care. A rapid reassessment on arrival at the receiving hospital would still be appropriate as it is difficult to examine a patient in a moving ambulance (or helicopter) and changes in the patient's condition may have been missed.

Better a negative laparotomy than a positive post mortem

The reason

If a patient remains hypotensive despite fluid resuscitation, the possibility of undetected intra-abdominal haemorrhage should be considered. No investigation is perfect and a negative diagnostic peritoneal lavage or abdominal CT scan should not dissuade the surgeon from performing a laparotomy in a deteriorating patient.

The exceptions

It is important to have excluded hidden blood loss into other body compartments (see Rule 18).

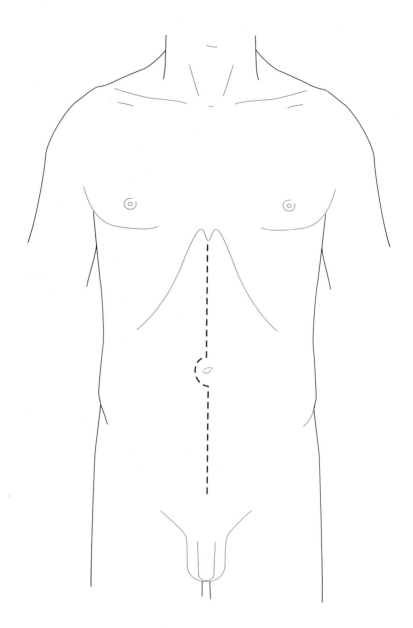

A midline incision.

Go down the middle and be liberal

The reason

A midline incision provides good access to all abdominal and pelvic structures and can be extended into the chest as a thoracotomy or median sternotomy. A laparotomy is the only intervention that will salvage a patient with exsanguinating intra-abdominal haemorrhage, and it can be performed in the operating theatre by any surgeon with basic experience. A senior surgeon should be summoned, but time should not be wasted while waiting for this surgeon to arrive.

Once the junior surgeon has opened the abdomen, free blood and clots should be rapidly evacuated and haemorrhage temporarily tamponaded. Tamponade is achieved by packing the left upper quadrant around the spleen, packing the right upper quadrant around and beneath the liver, applying a haemostat to a free bleeder in the messentry or mescolon, and packing the pelvic cavity if a large retroperitoneal haematoma is present. Immediate efforts should not be made to identify and arrest haemmhorage. These strategies can allow time for further transfusion and the arrival of a senior colleague. The definitive control of bleeding can then proceed in a more controlled fashion.

The exceptions

When dealing with a stab wound to the abdomen of a stable patient, it is appropriate to first perform a laparoscopy through a separate sub-umbilical incision to observe if the peritoneum is breached. If it is not breached then the wound can be explored and repaired. If the peritoneum is breached then a laparotomy is required, irrespective of other laparoscopic findings.

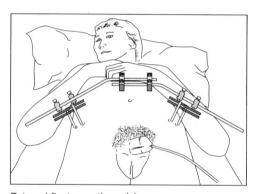

External fixator on the pelvis.

Fix the pelvis to fix the bleeding

The reason

The pelvis has a rich blood supply. Major blood vessels are in intimate contact with the pelvic bones. A displaced pelvic ring fracture may result in tearing of these vessels, and specifically the iliac vessels, with resultant life-threatening haemorrhage. By reducing and fixing the fracture the bleeding may be tamponaded.

To be accurate, pelvic stabilisation is particularly recommended for the group of patients who have a contained haematoma and who have sustained hypotension despite fluid resuscitation. Over 60% of patients with haemorrhage from unstable pelvic fractures will respond to fluid resuscitation alone, without the need for an external fixator, because the inherent natural boundaries of the pelvis result in spontaneous tamponade.[1] In those patients where a pelvic haematoma ruptures intraperitoneally, haemorrhage is often fatal.[2]

If a laparotomy is required the pelvis should be fixed before the incision, otherwise the tamponade is released without further bleeding being controlled and haemorrhage may be fatal.

The pelvis is stabilised with an external fixator or, in the short term, with Military Anti-Shock Trousers (Pneumatic Anti-Shock Garment).

The exceptions

Fixation may not be enough to stop the bleeding, and angiography with embolisation may be required.

[1]Flint L. Definitive control of bleeding from severe pelvic fractures. *Annals of Surgery* 1979; **189**: 709.
[2]Mucha P, Farnell M. Analysis of pelvic fracture management. *Journal of Trauma* 1984; **24**: 379.

Biology is the mother of all fixation

The reason

When a bone breaks, the natural biological process is that the broken ends will unite and heal. The more surgical interference there is with a fracture, the more interference there is with bone healing. Specifically, over-rigid fixation will reduce the ability of bone to heal.

Correction of malalignment, rotation, and shortening are all important for long-bone fractures, and fixation should be stable but not rigid.

The exceptions

As near perfect and rigid immobilisation as possible is recommended for intra-articular fractures and for those fractures of the adult forearm which, if inadequately treated, may interfere with pronation and supination.

The solution to pollution is dilution*

The reason

The main solution to contamination (pollution) of a wound is copious irrigation (dilution) rather than antibiotics. The solution used, whether it is sterile water or normal saline, is not critical as it is not absorbed, but it should be warmed to body temperature.

The irrigating solution is best delivered directly from the end of a giving set connected to the bag of fluid. Ten litres of fluid may be used to irrigate an open long-bone fracture.

The exceptions

The life-threatening complications of a wound must be dealt with before a wound toilet. Dirty and non-viable tissue will be removed rather than just irrigated.

* This rule is believed to be first attributed to Dr Mike Chapman, Surgeon, Texas, USA.

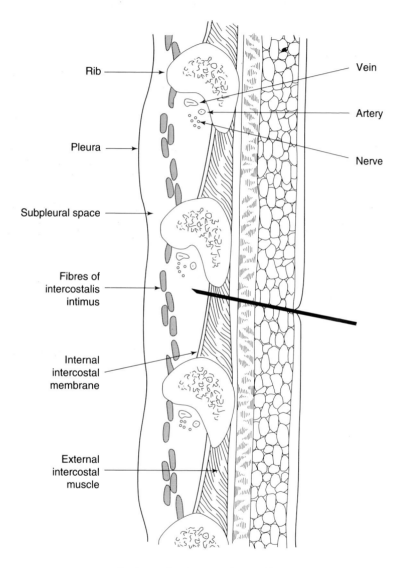

Anatomy of an intercostal nerve block.

(Modified from Nunn JA, Slavin G. *Br J Anaesth* **52**: 253-260, 1980.)

It doesn't pay to be complacent about an elderly fracture of the rib

The reason

Rib fractures are very painful, and if such an injury is sustained by an elderly patient, a heavy smoker, or a patient with existing chronic bronchitis then the pain may be enough to prevent the patient from clearing secretions by coughing. Fatal pneumonia can develop rapidly.

Always consider admitting such patients for analgesia and chest physiotherapy. Analgesic options include intercostal local anaesthetic nerve blocks and Patient Controlled Analgesia (PCA) systems.

These patients will typically deteriorate slowly over two to three days unless pain is relieved adequately and physiotherapy started. The aim must be to avoid intubation and IPPV (intermittent positive-pressure ventilation), with all its complications, if possible.

Remember that more ribs may be fractured than are evident on the chest x-ray.

The exceptions

Young and otherwise fit patients with no underlying pulmonary disease can be managed as outpatients with oral analgesia.

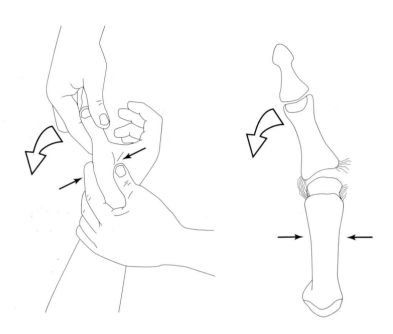

Examination of the ulna collateral ligament of the thumb.
Such a 'minor' problem can be easily missed in the
resuscitation room, but is potentially disabling.

A missed tertiary survey is a missed injury

The reason

The primary survey will discover life-threatening injuries compromising the airway, breathing, and circulation. The secondary survey will identify obvious injuries in each body region. Both of these surveys are performed under time pressure in the emergency department.

The tertiary survey is a repeated head-to-toe examination which will often discover minor injuries (and sometimes major injuries) missed in the emergency department. This is particularly true for minor fractures or ligament injuries. Its importance is that these "minor" orthopaedic problems can be the main cause of long-term disability. The tertiary survey is performed at leisure after life-saving surgery or the principal trauma radiological investigations and can be done in the emergency department, the intensive care unit, or the ward.

The exceptions

There are no exceptions. It costs nothing to examine a patient. A missed tertiary survey is a missed injury. So look, look again ... and look once more.

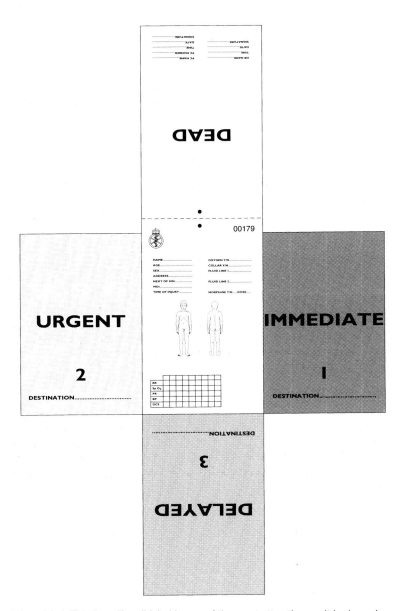

Triage label. This "cruciform" label is one of the most attractive, as it is dynamic and has adequate space for patient information.

With multiple casualties do the most for the most

The reason

When you are confronted with multiple casualties you must prioritise the injured for treatment. This is triage. The standard triage priorities are as follows:

IMMEDIATE	Requires immediate treatment, e.g. obstructed airway or tension pneumothorax
URGENT	Requires treatment within four hours, e.g. compound long-bone fracture
DELAYED	Can wait more than four hours for treatment, e.g. minor cuts and sprains
DEAD	

During the process of triage it will become obvious that there are some patients who will die even with the best available treatment. If medical resources are used for this casualty then others who were salvageable may also die. The decision to "do the most for the most" then becomes important, and those who will certainly die are labelled EXPECTANT and are left untreated.[1] This can be a very difficult decision as it is a reversal of normal health care priorities.

The exceptions

The EXPECTANT category is not invoked routinely at every multiple casualty incident but only when the medical resources are overwhelmed. At the incident site it will be a joint decision of the Medical Incident Officer (Medical Commander) and the Ambulance Incident Officer (Ambulance Commander) to invoke this triage category.

[1]Hodgetts T, Mackway-Jones K. *Major Incident Medical Management and Support: The practical approach.* London: BMJ Publishing Group, 1995.

Rule 58

Black is beautiful, and some things are never as black as they seem

The reason

When "dry gangrene" develops following non-freezing cold injury, the skin (often of the fingers or toes) appears black and dead. The depth of tissue necrosis in non-freezing cold is, however, often overestimated by the inexperienced observer who may wrongly assume that necrosis of the skin implies necrosis of deep tissues. This lack of understanding has led to unnecessary and inappropriately high amputations.

Surgical debridement or amputation following non-freezing cold injury should be delayed until the level of mummification is clearly demarcated, at around one to three months.[1]

The exceptions

"Wet gangrene" implies underlying infection. This is a surgical priority and requires immediate aggressive debridement, together with antibiotics.

[1]Fischer R, Souba W, Ford E. Temperature-associated injuries and syndromes. In: Moore E, Mattox K, Feliciano D. *Trauma*. Connecticut: Appleton and Lange, 1991.

Rehabilitation begins at the roadside

The reason

Up to 39% of pre-hospital trauma deaths result from simple treatable causes such as hypoxia and hypovolaemia and can be avoidable[1]. Avoidable deaths occur in hospital for the same reasons. Good pre-hospital care and hospital resuscitation may reduce mortality and, theoretically, will reduce morbidity, for example with a closed head injury:

- Clearing airway at the scene reduces secondary brain damage from hypoxia.
- Blood replacement in hospital reduces secondary brain damage from hypovolaemia.
- Early surgery to remove an extradural haematoma reduces secondary brain damage from pressure effects.

Recently, scientific evidence has questioned fluid resuscitation given pre-hospital or in the emergency department. Specifically, in hypotensive patients with penetrating torso injuries, there is an increased mortality in those patients who receive immediate fluid resuscitation compared to those whose resuscitation is delayed until arrival in the operating room.[2]

The exceptions

Prevention makes rehabilitation unnecessary. Innovations in road accident injury prevention have included:

- Speed restrictions
- Drink-driving legislation
- Front and rear seat-belts
- Airbags
- Side impact protection bars

[1]Hussain L, Redmond A. Are pre-hospital deaths from accidental injury preventable. *BMJ* 1994; **308**: 1077–80.
[2]Bickell W, Wall M, Pepe P, *et al.* Immediate versus delayed fluid resuscitation for hypotensive patients with penetrating torso injuries. *NEJM* 1994; **331**: 1105–9.

Death is the only certainty in life

The reason

Trauma is the biggest killer of children and adults under 35 years old in the developed world. A systematic team approach to trauma will help to reduce this mortality and the morbidity from serious injury. Some people will still die despite our best efforts.

This does not mean that we have failed. It does mean that we should continue to try hard to develop our trauma system and look for new ways to improve the outcome from trauma.

The exceptions

There are, unfortunately, none.

However, these rules **are** immortalised, and they may help you to save a life or two.

Reader's Rules

Use this space to note your own Trauma Rules.

If you wish to submit your rule(s) for inclusion in a future edition please send them to:

> BMJ Publishing Group
> BMA House
> Tavistock Square
> London
> WC1H 9JR

All contributions will be appropriately acknowledged.

Index

Index